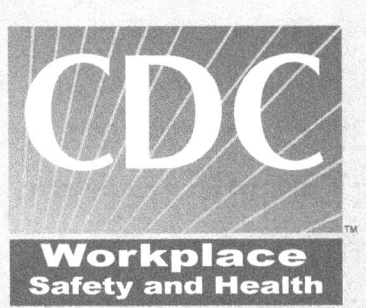

I0426168

Evaluation of Exposures Associated with Cleaning and Maintaining Composting Toilets – Arizona

Nancy Clark Burton, PhD, MPH, CIH
Chad Dowell, MS, CIH

Health Hazard Evaluation Report
HETA 2009-0100-3135
July 2011

DEPARTMENT OF HEALTH AND HUMAN SERVICES
Centers for Disease Control and Prevention

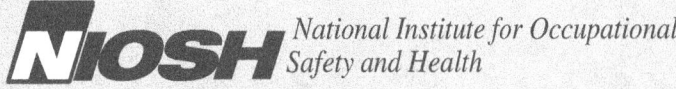

National Institute for Occupational Safety and Health

The employer shall post a copy of this report for a period of 30 calendar days at or near the workplace(s) of affected employees. The employer shall take steps to insure that the posted determinations are not altered, defaced, or covered by other material during such period. [37 FR 23640, November 7, 1972, as amended at 45 FR 2653, January 14, 1980].

CONTENTS

ABBREVIATIONS

ACGIH®	American Conference of Governmental Industrial Hygienists
CDC	Centers for Disease Control and Prevention
CL	Ceiling limit
CFR	Code of Federal Regulations
HAV	Hepatitis A virus
HBV	Hepatitis B virus
HHE	Health hazard evaluation
HPS	Hantavirus pulmonary syndrome
IDLH	Immediately dangerous to life or health
LFL	Lower flammable limit
ND	Not detected
NAICS	North American Industry Classification System
NIOSH	National Institute for Occupational Safety and Health
OEL	Occupational exposure limit
OSHA	Occupational Safety and Health Administration
PAPR	Powered air-purifying respirator
PBZ	Personal breathing zone
PPE	Personal protective equipment
PEL	Permissible exposure limit
ppm	Parts per million
REL	Recommended exposure limit
STEL	Short-term exposure limit
TLV®	Threshold limit value
TWA	Time-weighted average
U.S. EPA	United States Environmental Protection Agency
WEEL™	Workplace environmental exposure level

The National Institute for Occupational Safety and Health (NIOSH) received a request for a health hazard evaluation at a national park in Arizona. Management submitted the request because of concerns about exposures to employees cleaning and maintaining pit and composting toilets. The request also asked for an evaluation of personal protective equipment (PPE) use.

What NIOSH Did

- We visited the park in May 2009.

- We talked with management and employees about their concerns.

- We observed employee work practices and PPE use.

- We reviewed the park's written respiratory protection program. We also reviewed material safety data sheets for cleaners and bacteria additives used at the park.

- We collected personal breathing zone and area air samples for ammonia, hydrogen sulfide, enteric bacteria (as an indicator of fecal contamination), and thermophilic actinomycetes (as an indicator of the microbial contamination found at the higher temperatures needed to compost organic material).

What NIOSH Found

- Ammonia concentrations were higher when the pit toilets were opened than when the composting toilets were opened. These concentrations dropped quickly when the ammonia was exposed to air.

- Air sampling showed that thermophilic bacteria were present when the employees worked with the composting toilets.

- Hydrogen sulfide and enteric bacteria were not found in air samples.

- Work tasks required manual shoveling and lifting and some awkward postures.

- Working in the park puts employees at risk for extreme heat, bee and scorpion stings, spider bites, and hantavirus from rodent nests and feces.

- Employees may be exposed to hepatitis A virus (HAV) when handling untreated human waste and trash. Employees may also be exposed to hepatitis B virus (HAB) while doing other job duties as first responders.

What Managers Can Do

- Use metal supports to allow the contents of the pit toilets to be dumped directly into the storage container for disposal.

- Increase how often preventive maintenance is performed on toilets. This will allow issues such as blocked leachate lines to be identified and addressed more quickly.

- Include trail maintenance crews in current bloodborne pathogen program, and require employees to take annual training.

- Start a voluntary vaccination program for HAV and HBV for the trail and toilet maintenance crews.

- Develop standard medical follow-up protocols for bee and scorpion stings and spider bites.

- Implement a confined space program. This program should be followed when entering and emptying the composting toilet vaults.

- Start a heat stress program for the trail and toilet maintenance crews.

What Employees Can Do

- Wear the right PPE for the work you are doing including gloves, protective clothing, and NIOSH-approved respirator.

- Clean your hands before eating, drinking, or smoking.

- Wait 1 minute after opening the lid of a pit toilet before servicing. This will allow the ammonia levels to dissipate.

- Seek prompt medical care for scorpion stings, bee stings, and spider bites.

- Get vaccinated for HAV if working with toilets and for HBV if your job involves first aid.

SUMMARY

NIOSH evaluated exposures to park employees who cleaned and maintained pit and composting toilets. We found that employees who serviced the pit and composting toilets were potentially exposed to a wide range of hazards. Identified hazards included exposure to infectious agents, chemicals, wildlife, and ergonomic stressors and working in hot environments and confined spaces. Engineering, administrative, and PPE recommendations to reduce these exposures such as using a backhoe to dump pit toilets into a dumpster and establishing a heat stress program are included in this report.

In February 2009, NIOSH received an HHE request from management at a national park in Arizona. The request concerned employees' potential exposures during the cleaning and maintenance of the pit and composting toilets in the park. Park management also wanted to know whether the PPE used by employees was appropriate. NIOSH investigators visited the park in May 2009. We held an opening meeting to discuss employer and employee concerns; observed work practices; talked to employees about their work and health; reviewed records; and collected air samples for ammonia, hydrogen sulfide, enteric bacteria, and thermophilic actinomycetes.

Our investigation showed that instantaneous ammonia concentrations were highest when the pit toilets were first opened, but these levels dropped very quickly. Thermophilic actinomycetes, an indicator of the microbial contamination found at the higher temperatures needed to compost organic material, were detected in PBZ air samples collected while employees cleaned composting toilets. No hydrogen sulfide or enteric bacteria were detected. Heat stress was not evaluated during this site visit but could be a potential problem on the basis of ambient temperatures, workload, and use of PPE observed.

Other potential exposures for employees included scorpion and bee stings, spider bites, and airborne hantavirus from rodent nests and rodent feces. Employees were also potentially exposed to hepatitis A and hepatitis B viruses through first responder duties and through handling of untreated human waste and feminine hygiene products. Shoveling out the toilets by hand resulted in awkward postures. One of the composting toilets had a blocked leachate line that caused liquid to back up into the waste vault. Working inside the composting toilet vault meets the criteria for a confined space under NIOSH guidelines. Recommendations to address these potential hazards, such as development of standard medical procedures to address scorpion and bee stings and spider bites, are included in this report.

Keywords: NAICS 712190 (Nature Parks and Other Similar Institutions), composting toilets, pit toilets, sewage, enteric bacteria, thermophilic actinomycetes, confined space, ammonia, personal protective equipment

This page left intentionally blank

INTRODUCTION

On February 20, 2009, NIOSH received an HHE request from management at a national park in Arizona. The request was submitted because employees were concerned about exposures to human waste and wanted to know the appropriate PPE to use while cleaning and maintaining the three types of toilets used on the trails. NIOSH investigators conducted a site visit from May 12–15, 2009. An interim letter was sent in June 2009 with preliminary recommendations.

ASSESSMENT

We observed work processes, work practices, workplace conditions, and PPE use and spoke with employees about their potential exposures and health concerns. We reviewed the scientific literature concerning composting toilets and exposures associated with sewage. We also reviewed material safety data sheets for cleaning chemicals, standard operating procedures, and the written respiratory protection program. Dräger® short-term colorimetric detection tubes were used to measure airborne concentrations of ammonia and hydrogen sulfide when opening the toilets [Dräger Safety Inc., Pittsburgh, Pennsylvania]. The ammonia tubes have a standard measurement range of 5 to 100 ppm during a 10-second sampling period, and the hydrogen sulfide tubes have a range of 2 to 200 ppm during a 3.5-minute sampling period [Dräger 2011].

Task-based PBZ and area air samples were collected using a 0.3-micrometer pore-size 37-millimeter polytetrafluoroethylene filter in conjunction with an SKC AirChek 2000 sampling pump at a flow rate of 2 liters per minute (SKC Inc., Eighty Four, Pennsylvania). Samples were collected during pit and composting toilet cleaning and were analyzed for culturable enteric bacteria and culturable thermophilic actinomycetes (composting toilet cleaning only). An additional area air sample for enteric bacteria and thermophilic actinomycetes was collected below the composting toilets along the major trail. All sampling pumps were precalibrated and postcalibrated with a DryCal DC Lite (Bios International Corporation, Butler, New Jersey). Additional information regarding relevant OELs and health effects can be found in Appendix A.

Process Observations

Two groups of employees were potentially exposed – the compost crew and the rangers/trail crews. The compost crew cleaned the toilets and removed excess material in all three types of toilets used in the park – Romtec (pit), Phoenix (composting), and Clivus (composting). Maintenance of the pit toilets, performed by both groups of employees, included stirring the piles; general cleaning of the units using Simple Green®, a detergent solution containing 2-butoxyethanol; removing trash from the toilets; and restocking of supplies. PPE used for maintenance included latex or nitrile gloves, rubber outer gloves, and safety glasses. Alcohol hand wash (62% ethanol) was used for hand cleaning. General maintenance of the trail composting toilets included replacing toilet paper, adding wood chips and sewage treatment bacteria, sweeping floors and cleaning surfaces, removing trash and replacing trash can liners, mopping floors, and stirring and raking the toilet contents. This work was done by the composting crew and the rangers/trail crews.

The Romtec units were used in the back country. These units were loaded onto large metal trays and flown in and out of the park by helicopter. Cleaning out the Romtec units consisted of removing the wet material and wood chips from the base with a shovel and putting them into a backhoe (Figure 1). The backhoe operator moved the wet material and wood chips to a large trailer where they were mixed in with other trash before being taken to an off-site municipal landfill. The compost crew wore nitrile gloves under rubber gloves, work boots, goggles, Tyvek® suit, and a facemask (Defend Model MK-1006). The employees voluntarily used facemasks to keep flies out of their noses and mouths rather than for respiratory protection. We noticed leakage from the backhoe's split claw into the dirt pit when the employees shoveled out the Romtec toilets, potentially exposing them to untreated waste.

The large and heavy Romtec units were loaded onto a truck by two employees and driven to the wastewater treatment plant where they were scrubbed using brushes with a Simple Green® detergent solution (Sunshine Makers, Inc., Huntington Harbour, California), rinsed with water, and sanitized with a hypochlorite solution (1½ cups of household bleach in 1 gallon of water) (Figure 2). The employees wore rubber waders over Tyvek suits, rubber boots, nitrile gloves under rubber gloves, and facemasks (Defend Model MK-1006).

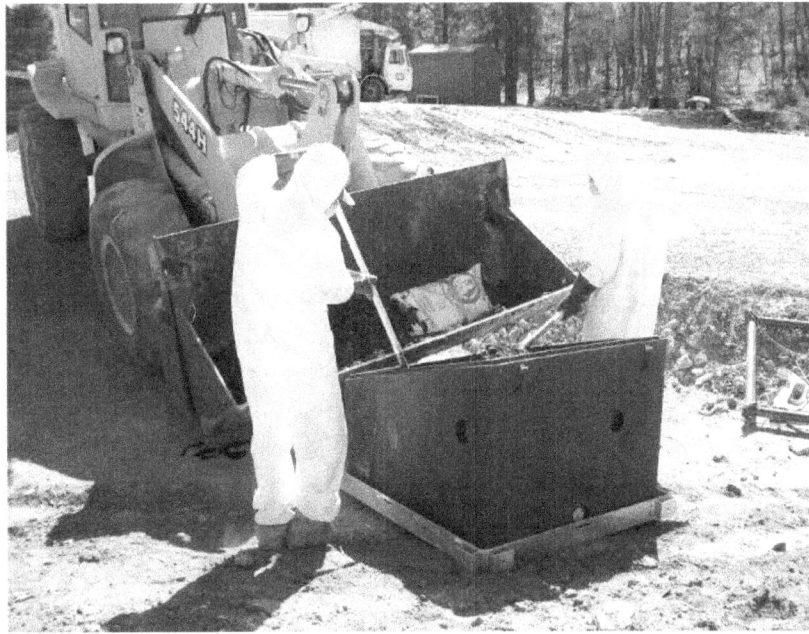

Figure 1. Employees in PPE shoveling material from a pit toilet into a backhoe clamshell shovel.

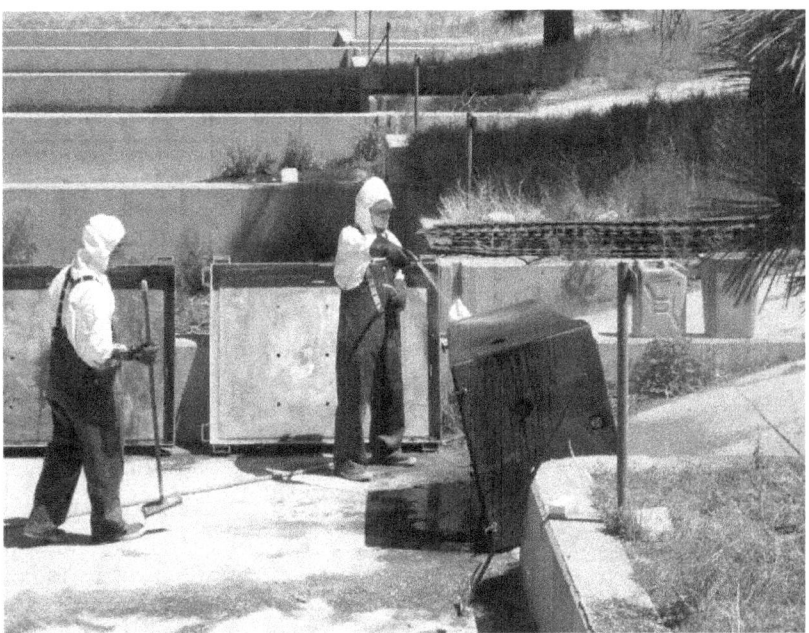

Figure 2. Employees in PPE cleaning pit toilet components at the wastewater treatment plant.

The Phoenix and Clivus composting toilets were designed to break down waste materials using naturally occurring bacteria and fungi and supplemental bacteria, which is added during toilet maintenance. A composting toilet is divided into an upper section for public use and below-ground composting tanks (Figure 3). The waste was turned using either solar battery-powered or wired electrical baffles. At least annually the composting crew removed the waste from the composting toilets. To prevent exposure to hantavirus, the crew used a hypochlorite solution (1½ cups of household bleach in 1 gallon of water) in the lower section of the composting tanks if rodent droppings were present. Most of the work was shoveling the waste into bags (weight range: 36 to 74 pounds). The bags were carried out of the park by mule train and then taken to a landfill. During the NIOSH site visit, the compost crew wore latex or nitrile gloves under rubber gloves, work boots, Tyvek suits, and hooded 3M PAPRs with high efficiency particulate filters during active cleaning.

One of the composting toilets along the trail, installed in the 1980s, reportedly had a nonfunctioning leachate line that caused liquid to build up in the composting vaults. As a result, it was necessary to add several bags of wood chips to soak up the liquid before the vault could be emptied. The wet wood chips were heavy and hard to shovel (Figure 4).

Occasionally, some of the waste got stuck in the toilet's waste chute. To loosen the waste, the employee put his or her head and shoulders into the vault and used a shovel or a metal bar to dislodge the stuck waste. This vault was considered a confined space (Category C) under NIOSH definitions because it had a limited opening for entry and exit, unfavorable natural ventilation with potentially dangerous contaminants, and was not intended for continuous employee occupancy [NIOSH 1979]. The Phoenix toilets had a crank attached to baffles to help break up material so that it could fall into the vault. Employees reported that awkward postures and the weight of the material made it hard to shovel while squatting and filling bags (Figure 5). We observed that employees did not lock the upstairs doors, and untreated waste fell on them when people used the facilities. The outside of the bags had some waste stuck to them, which was difficult to remove and could contact the workers' and mules' skin.

The compost crew worked in pairs to move the Romtec equipment and the full bags of composting material. Both were heavy and awkward to handle.

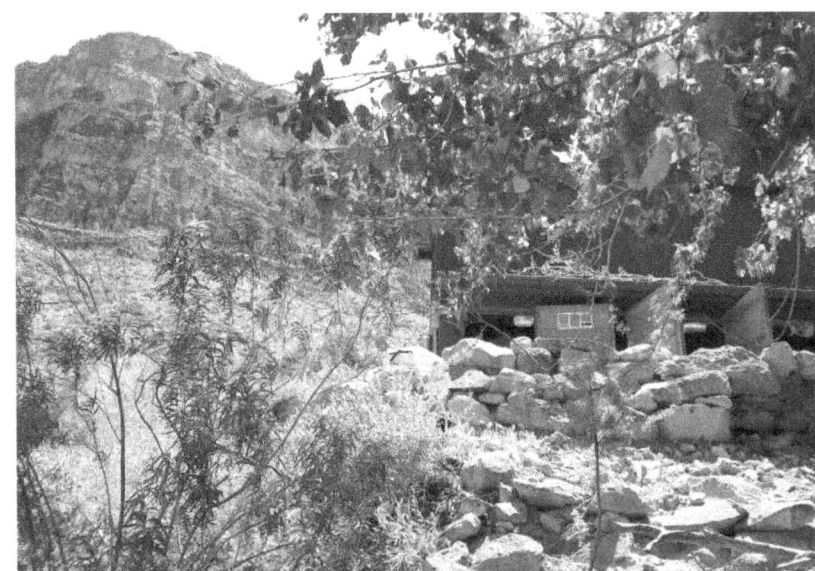

Figure 3. Bank of composting toilets on the trail.

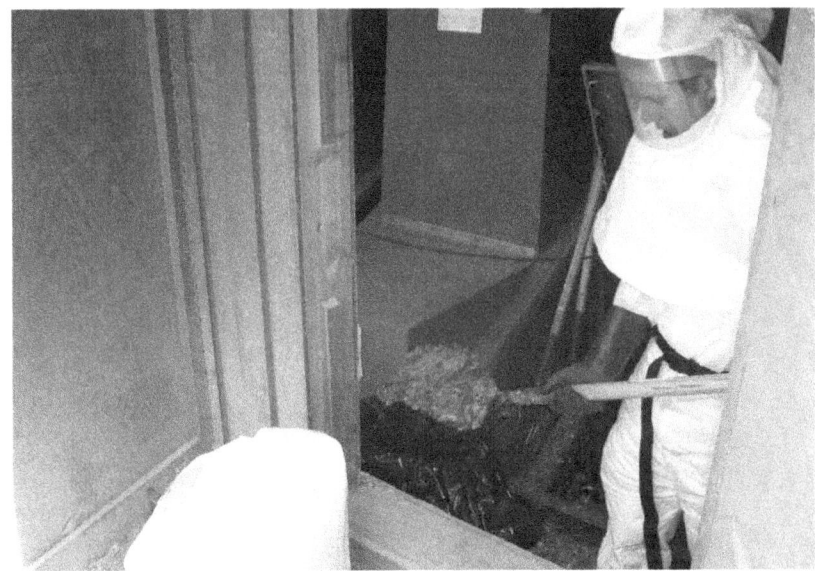

Figure 4. Employee wearing hooded PAPR shoveling wood chips saturated with liquid out of a composting toilet.

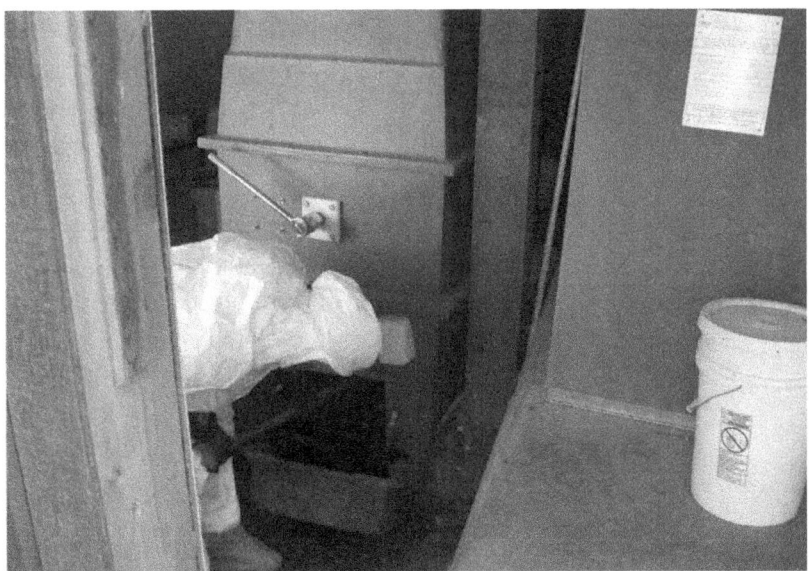

Figure 5. Employee in Tyvek clothing bending over to shovel out the vault of a composting toilet.

Park employees are potentially exposed to heat stress. Temperatures were over 120°F in the sun (park thermometer) during the site visit; few areas of shade were available. Wearing PPE added to the heat burden. The crew took frequent breaks and rehydrated with water during these breaks.

We talked to employees about the hazards associated with wildlife that could live in and around the pit and composting toilets. Wildlife encountered in the past included black widow spiders, scorpions, and rodents. We saw a scorpion in the carrying tray of one of the Romtec units. Flies came out of the Romtec toilet when the lid was opened. We observed maggots all over the seat after the lid was left open during the cleaning process.

The employees expressed concern over potential exposures to HAV and HBV. The compost crew was vaccinated for both exposures, the rangers were vaccinated for HBV, and the trail crew was vaccinated for neither. All employees received tetanus vaccinations.

The employees explained that the trail crew provided first aid to park visitors and fellow employees when needed until additional staff arrived on the scene of an emergency. These emergencies included cuts and broken bones from falls. They expressed concern that they were not included in the vaccination program.

Air Sampling

Area ammonia and hydrogen sulfide concentrations are presented in Table 1. When we first opened the Romtec pit toilets, ammonia levels were high (50 ppm and 70 ppm); however, the levels quickly dropped when exposed to the ambient air. The ammonia levels probably did not exceed the NIOSH and ACGIH STEL of 35 ppm for a 15-minute air sample, because these were instantaneous air samples. No hydrogen sulfide was detected at a limit of detection of 2 ppm.

No enteric bacteria were detected in the air samples (Table 2). Thermophilic actinomycetes, Gram-positive organisms found in soil and composting material, were detected in PBZ air samples from employees performing maintenance tasks on the Clivus and Phoenix composting toilets and in the area air sample collected below the composting toilets. No OELs have been established for either of these microbial agents.

Table 1. Direct reading air samples for ammonia and hydrogen sulfide

Activity	Ammonia (ppm)*	Hydrogen Sulfide (ppm)
Opening Romtec 1 toilet seat lid	70	ND†
Opening Romtec 2 toilet seat lid	50	ND
Opening bottom bin of Clivus composting toilet	ND	ND
Opening top of Phoenix toilet inside lower area	4	ND

*ppm—parts per million
†Not detected above the limit of detection (ammonia: 5 ppm; hydrogen sulfide: 2 ppm)

Table 2. Qualitative task-based and area air sampling results for enteric bacteria and thermophilic actinomycetes

Activity	Sampling Time	Enteric Bacteria	Thermophilic Actinomycetes
Opening/shoveling out Romtec toilet	8:20 a.m.–9:41 a.m.	ND*	†
Opening/shoveling out Romtec toilet	8:21 a.m.–9:41 a.m.	ND	†
Cleaning out Romtec toilet at wastewater treatment plant	10:21 a.m.–11:41 a.m.	ND	†
Cleaning out Romtec toilet at wastewater treatment plant	10:21 a.m.–11:42 a.m.	ND	†
Maintenance/shoveling out Clivus toilet	8:20 a.m.–9:41 a.m.	ND	ND
Maintenance/shoveling out Phoenix toilet	8:20 a.m.–9:41 a.m.	ND	ND
Maintenance on Clivus toilet/ carrying and weighing bags	12:16 p.m.–2:57 p.m.	ND	‡
Maintenance on Phoenix toilet/ carrying and weighing bags	12:16 p.m.–2:55 p.m.	ND	‡
Area sample–shelter	12:18 p.m.–2:59 p.m.	ND	‡

*ND—not detected
†Not analyzed (too wet)
‡Positive culture for bacteria

DISCUSSION

The park has approximately 4.5 million visitors a year, which makes the maintenance of the toilet facilities important for public health and environmental impact reasons [NPS 2010]. Composting toilets have been available commercially for about 40 years [U.S. EPA 1999]. Composting toilets treat pathogens to reduce the risk of infection and avoid environmental contamination. Four major types of human pathogenic organisms are found in human waste: (1) bacteria, (2) viruses, (3) protozoa, and (4) helminths (parasitic worms) [U.S. EPA 2003; Arthurson 2008]. The amount of pathogens present depends on the initial concentration and the amount of physical and biological decomposition that has occurred. The composting operation uses time, temperature, and aeration to facilitate the decomposition process [Arthurson 2008].

The moisture level in the composting toilets needed to be controlled for the composting process to produce usable compost. All but one of the composting toilets along the trail was functioning as designed. The malfunctioning toilet had a blocked leachate line, which allowed liquid to accumulate in the vault. This affected the composting process and made cleaning the vault more difficult. The composting crew had to add wood chips to the vault, which increased the weight and volume. Cleaning the vault occasionally required crew members to enter the vault up to their chest; therefore, this area met the NIOSH definition of a confined space.

The cleaning process for both types of toilets was labor intensive, requiring hand shoveling into either a backhoe loader or into bags, loading and unloading of pit toilets into a truck to take them to final cleaning, and manual carrying of the filled bags of waste to the mule station. Employees were potentially exposed to human waste when cleaning both types of toilets. Contact with the material on the tools used to remove the waste (shovels and/or metal bar) and with the outside of the bags were potential venues for exposure. Activities such as walking through wet material and keeping the toilets in service during the maintenance process also provided potential exposure, as did the flies landing on the employees after they had landed on the bags and raw sewage.

Our review of the scientific literature shows that the occupational exposure assessments for composting sewage sludge have focused on large municipal operations [Clark et al. 1983; Clark et al. 1984; Johanning 1999; NIOSH 1999a,b,c; Schlosser et al. 2009]. Documented exposures for these activities included exposure to ammonia, thermophilic actinomycetes, Gram negative and *Bacillus* bacteria, endotoxin, and fungal genera (*Cladosporium, Aspergillus,* and *Penicillium*). We found potential exposures to ammonia and thermophilic actinomycetes in this evaluation. Enteric bacteria were not found in our task-based PBZ air sampling.

The PPE used by the employees was appropriate for the work that was being performed but may have increased the risk of heat stress. The written respiratory protection policy was comprehensive, including training, medical clearance, and fit testing in accordance with OSHA requirements under 29 CFR 1910.134. However, it did not specifically mention the use of the loose-fitting PAPR for the compost toilet maintenance work. The PAPRs had been purchased just before the NIOSH site visit. The written policy stated that an N100 filtering facepiece respirator should be worn while cleaning the composting toilets because of the potential for exposure to hantavirus, but CDC guidelines state that workers should use either a negative-pressure half-face air purifying respirator with N100 or P100 filters or a PAPR with high efficiency particulate filters [Mills et al. 2002]. We observed employees wearing only a facemask, not a respirator. Facemasks provided barrier protection against flies but are not considered respiratory protection.

While cleaning and maintaining toilets, employees had the potential for exposure to spiders, scorpions, and rodents/nesting material that could contain hantavirus. Employees also had a potential for exposure to HAV from handling the untreated waste in the pit toilets and to HBV from handling the trash (mostly feminine hygiene products) and from conducting first responder duties. More detailed information on the health issues associated with these exposures is provided in Appendix A.

CONCLUSIONS

Employees who cleaned and serviced the pit and composting toilets were potentially exposed to a wide range of hazards including infectious agents, chemicals, heat, confined space, ergonomic stressors, and wildlife. We measured elevated ammonia levels when opening the Romtec toilets, but the levels rapidly dropped when diluted with outdoor air. We found that employees were exposed to airborne thermophilic actinomycetes, which can cause inflammatory lung disease, when cleaning out the composting toilets. The employees also had a potential for exposure to scorpion stings, spider bites, and airborne hantavirus from rodent nests/feces. Potential exposure to bloodborne pathogens, such as HAV and HBV from handling untreated human waste and when performing first aid, was also a concern.

RECOMMENDATIONS

On the basis of our findings, we recommend the actions listed below to create a more healthful workplace. We encourage park management to use a labor-management health and safety committee or working group to discuss the recommendations in this report and develop an action plan. Those involved in the work can best set priorities and assess the feasibility of our recommendations for the specific situation at the park. Our recommendations are based on the hierarchy of controls approach (Appendix A: Occupational Exposure Limits and Health Effects). This approach groups actions by their likely effectiveness in reducing or removing hazards. In most cases, the preferred approach is to eliminate hazardous materials or processes and install engineering controls to reduce exposure or shield employees. Until such controls are in place, or if they are not effective or feasible, administrative measures and/or personal protective equipment may be needed.

Engineering Controls

Engineering controls reduce exposures to employees by removing the hazard from the process or placing a barrier between the hazard and the employee. Engineering controls are very effective at protecting employees without placing primary responsibility of implementation on the employee.

1. Develop a new method for emptying the Romtec toilets such as adding supports to the bottom of the Romtec container and using the backhoe to dump it into the landfill storage container. This will reduce exposures to untreated human waste and ergonomic hazards among the compost crew.

2. Replace or unblock the leachate lines for the trail toilets by clearing with a plumbing snake, using a pump to remove the liquid material, or installing a new evaporator system like the one used in the newer toilets. This will facilitate the composting process, reduce exposure to liquid waste, and minimize ergonomic hazards.

3. Design future toilet facilities with adequate space to allow the crew room to service them (manually remove waste) from the basement level.

Administrative Controls

Administrative controls are management-dictated work practices and policies to reduce or prevent exposures to workplace hazards. The effectiveness of administrative changes in work practices for controlling workplace hazards is dependent on management commitment and employee acceptance. Regular monitoring and reinforcement are necessary to ensure that control policies and procedures are not circumvented in the name of convenience or production.

1. Implement an administrative policy to open the Romtec toilets and have the employees move away from the area for a brief period (such as 1 minute) to reduce exposure to ammonia. Because this work is done outdoors, the ammonia levels are diluted quickly.

2. Develop a confined space policy for entering the composting toilet vault. It meets the NIOSH criterion for a confined space, and all relevant NIOSH guidelines for such confined spaces should be adhered to when entry is made into the composting toilet vault to pull down excess material (Appendix B). This includes using the checklist of considerations for entry, working in, and exiting confined spaces. Additional information can be found at http://www.cdc.gov/niosh/topics/confinedspace/.

3. Encourage employees to always wash their hands with soap and water, if available, or use hand sanitizer after removing gloves and before eating, drinking, or smoking.

4. Increase the number of times preventive maintenance on the toilet systems is done each year to prevent problems from developing and to reduce the amount of physical labor needed to clean the toilets [U.S. EPA 1999]. This allows problems such as blocked leachate lines to be identified and addressed in a timelier manner.

5. Follow the recommendations for preventing heat stress and strain as described in a prior NIOSH HHE report, especially the sections concerning administrative controls and heat strain monitoring. This report can be found at http://www.cdc.gov/niosh/hhe/reports/pdfs/1999-0321-2873.pdf.

6. Implement a voluntary HAV vaccination program for the trail crew and rangers. Include trail crews in annual bloodborne pathogen training required by OSHA if they are going to perform first aid activities, and offer HBV vaccinations to the trail crews.

7. Follow the recommendations outlined in Appendix A for dealing with scorpion or bee stings or spider bites. Establish standard operating procedures to deal with scorpion or bee stings or spider bites, and provide first aid kits with appropriate supplies so employees can treat these stings or bites when out on the trails. Insect repellants can be used to reduce exposures to flies and other pests.

8. Set up a policy to take toilets out of service during maintenance procedures to avoid direct exposure to untreated human waste.

9. Use a sunscreen with a minimum skin protection factor of 15 to prevent exposure to ultraviolet radiation, which is a risk factor for sunburn and skin cancer.

Personal Protective Equipment

PPE is the least effective means for controlling employee exposures. Proper use of PPE requires a comprehensive program and calls for a high level of employee involvement and commitment to be effective. The use of PPE requires the choice of the appropriate equipment to reduce the hazard and the development of supporting programs such as training, change-out schedules, and medical assessment if needed. PPE should not be relied upon as the sole method for limiting employee exposures. Rather, PPE should be used until engineering and administrative controls can be demonstrated to be effective in limiting exposures to acceptable levels.

1. Continue to use the current PPE when maintaining and cleaning the toilets.

2. Update the written respiratory protection policy to include the PAPRs, and establish cleaning and maintenance

Recommendations
(continued)

procedures on their use including the regular replacement of the hoods if contaminated with untreated waste.

3. Provide training on the use of PAPRs and their cleaning and maintenance.

4. Use yellow rubber boots over the compost crew's work boots to prevent the spread of contamination when work boots get wet.

5. Use protective gloves made of synthetic latex, vinyl, or nitrile. The latex gloves provide an effective barrier against biological agents, but because the use of natural latex poses a risk for developing latex allergy, other gloves should be used [NIOSH 1999d].

References

Arthurson V [2008]. Proper sanitization of sewage sludge: a critical issue for a sustainable society. Appl Environ Microbiol 74(17):5267–5275.

Clark CS, Bjornson HS, Schwartz-Fulton J, Holland JW, Gartside PS [1984]. Biological health risks associated with the composting of wastewater treatment plant sludge. J Water Pollut Control Fed 56(12):1269–1276.

Clark CS, Rylander R, Larsson l [1983]. Levels of Gram-negative bacteria, *Aspergillus fumigatus*, dust, and endotoxin at compost plants. Appl Environ Microbiol 45(5):1501–1505.

Dräger [2010]. Short-term measurements with Dräger-Tubes. [http://www.draeger.com/US/en_US/]. Date accessed: June 2011.

Johanning E [1999]. An overview of waste management in the United States and recent research activities about composting related occupational health risk. Schriftenr Ver Wasser Boden Lufthyg 104:127–140.

Mills JN, Corneli A, Young JC, Garrison LE, Khan AS, Ksiazek TG [2002]. Hantavirus pulmonary syndrome–United States: updated recommendations for risk reduction. MMWR 51(RR-9) 1–12.

NPS [2010]. NP reports: annual park visitation. [http://www.nature.nps.gov/stats/viewReport.cfm]. Date accessed: June 2011.

REFERENCES
(CONTINUED)

NIOSH [1979]. Criteria for a recommended standard: Working in Confined Spaces. Cincinnati, OH: U.S. Department of Health, Education, and Welfare, Center for Disease Control, National Institute for Occupational Safety and Health, DHEW (NIOSH) Publication No. 80–106.

NIOSH [1999a]. Health hazard evaluation report: Central Maui Composting Facility Maui, Hawaii. By Burkhart JE. Morgantown, WV: U.S. Department of Health and Human Services, Centers for Disease Control and Prevention, National Institute for Occupational Safety and Health, NIOSH HETA No. 95-0203-2764.

NIOSH [1999b]. Health hazard evaluation report: City of Springfield, Department of Public Works Composting Facility, Springfield, Missouri. By Burkhart JE. Morgantown, WV: U.S. Department of Health and Human Services, Centers for Disease Control and Prevention, National Institute for Occupational Safety and Health, NIOSH HETA No. 95-0198-2765.

NIOSH [1999c]. Health hazard evaluation report: San Francisco Recreation and Parks Department, San Francisco, California. By Burkhart JE. Morgantown, WV: U.S. Department of Health and Human Services, Centers for Disease Control and Prevention, National Institute for Occupational Safety and Health, NIOSH HETA No. 95-0203-0252-2763.

NIOSH [1999d]. Latex allergy: a prevention guide. Cincinnati, OH: U.S. Department of Health and Human Services, Centers for Disease Control and Prevention, National Institute for Occupational Safety and Health, NIOSH Publication No. 98-113.

Schlosser O, Huyard A, Cartnick K, Yañez A, Catalán V, Quang ZD [2009]. Bioaerosol in composting facilities: occupational health risk assessment. .Water Environ Res 81(9):866–877.

U.S. EPA [1999]. Water efficiency technology fact sheet: composting toilets. Washington, DC: United States Environmental Protection Agency, Office of Water. EPA 832-F-99-066. [http://www.epa.gov/owm/mtb/comp.pdf]. Date accessed: June 2011.

U.S. EPA [2003]. Environmental regulations and technology— control of pathogens and vector attraction in sewage sludge. Washington, DC: Environmental Protection Agency, Office of Research and Development. EPA/625/R-92/013.

APPENDIX A: OCCUPATIONAL EXPOSURE LIMITS AND HEALTH EFFECTS

In evaluating the hazards posed by workplace exposures, NIOSH investigators use both mandatory (legally enforceable) and recommended OELs for chemical, physical, and biological agents as a guide for making recommendations. OELs have been developed by federal agencies and safety and health organizations to prevent the occurrence of adverse health effects from workplace exposures. Generally, OELs suggest levels of exposure that most employees may be exposed to for up to 10 hours per day, 40 hours per week, for a working lifetime, without experiencing adverse health effects. However, not all employees will be protected from adverse health effects even if their exposures are maintained below these levels. A small percentage may experience adverse health effects because of individual susceptibility, a preexisting medical condition, and/or hypersensitivity (allergy). In addition, some hazardous substances may act in combination with other workplace exposures, the general environment, or with medications or personal habits of the employee to produce adverse health effects even if the occupational exposures are controlled at the level set by the exposure limit. Also, some substances can be absorbed by direct contact with the skin and mucous membranes in addition to being inhaled, which contributes to the individual's overall exposure.

Most OELs are expressed as a TWA exposure. A TWA refers to the average exposure during a normal 8- to 10-hour workday. Some chemical substances and physical agents have recommended STEL or ceiling values where adverse health effects are caused by exposures over a short period. Unless otherwise noted, the STEL is a 15-minute TWA exposure that should not be exceeded at any time during a workday, and the CL is an exposure that should not be exceeded at any time.

In the United States, OELs have been established by federal agencies, professional organizations, state and local governments, and other entities. Some OELs are legally enforceable limits, while others are recommendations. The U.S. Department of Labor OSHA PELs (29 CFR 1910 [general industry]; 29 CFR 1926 [construction industry]; and 29 CFR 1917 [maritime industry]) are legal limits enforceable in workplaces covered under the Occupational Safety and Health Act of 1970. NIOSH RELs are recommendations based on a critical review of the scientific and technical information available on a given hazard and the adequacy of methods to identify and control the hazard. NIOSH RELs can be found in the *NIOSH Pocket Guide to Chemical Hazards* [NIOSH 2005]. NIOSH also recommends different types of risk management practices (e.g., engineering controls, safe work practices, employee education/ training, personal protective equipment, and exposure and medical monitoring) to minimize the risk of exposure and adverse health effects from these hazards. Other OELs that are commonly used and cited in the United States include the TLVs recommended by ACGIH, a professional organization, and the WEELs recommended by the American Industrial Hygiene Association, another professional organization. The TLVs and WEELs are developed by committee members of these associations from a review of the published, peer-reviewed literature. They are not consensus standards. ACGIH TLVs are considered voluntary exposure guidelines for use by industrial hygienists and others trained in this discipline "to assist in the control of health hazards" [ACGIH 2011]. WEELs have been established for some chemicals "when no other legal or authoritative limits exist" [AIHA 2010].

Outside the United States, OELs have been established by various agencies and organizations and include both legal and recommended limits. Since 2006, the Berufsgenossenschaftliches Institut für Arbeitsschutz (German Institute for Occupational Safety and Health) has maintained a database of international OELs from European Union member states, Canada (Québec), Japan, Switzerland, and the United States. The database, available at http://www.dguv.de/ifa/en/gestis/limit_values/index.jsp, contains international limits for over 1500 hazardous substances and is updated periodically.

Employers should understand that not all hazardous chemicals have specific OSHA PELs, and for some agents the legally enforceable and recommended limits may not reflect current health-based information. However, an employer is still required by OSHA to protect its employees from hazards even in the absence of a specific OSHA PEL. OSHA requires an employer to furnish employees a place of employment free from recognized hazards that cause or are likely to cause death or serious physical harm [Occupational Safety and Health Act of 1970 (Public Law 91–596, sec. 5(a)(1))]. Thus, NIOSH investigators encourage employers to make use of other OELs when making risk assessments and risk management decisions to best protect the health of their employees. NIOSH investigators also encourage the use of the traditional hierarchy of controls approach to eliminate or minimize identified workplace hazards. This includes, in order of preference, the use of (1) substitution or elimination of the hazardous agent, (2) engineering controls (e.g , local exhaust ventilation, process enclosure, dilution ventilation), (3) administrative controls (e.g., limiting time of exposure, employee training, work practice changes, medical surveillance), and (4) personal protective equipment (e.g., respiratory protection, gloves, eye protection, hearing protection). Control banding, a qualitative risk assessment and risk management tool, is a complementary approach to protecting employee health that focuses resources on exposure controls by describing how a risk needs to be managed. Information on control banding is available at http://www.cdc.gov/niosh/topics/ctrlbanding/. This approach can be applied in situations where OELs have not been established or can be used to supplement the OELs, when available.

Ammonia

Ammonia is a colorless, strongly alkaline, extremely soluble gas with a characteristic pungent odor. It is a severe irritant of the eyes, respiratory tract, and skin. Repeated exposure to ammonia vapor may cause chronic irritation of the eyes and upper respiratory tract [ATSDR 2004]. The NIOSH REL for ammonia is 25 ppm for a 10-hour TWA. The NIOSH STEL for ammonia is 35 ppm. The ACGIH has established a TLV of 25 ppm as an 8-hour TWA and a STEL of 35 ppm. The OSHA PEL for ammonia is 50 ppm for an 8-hour TWA.

Scorpions and Spiders

Scorpions mostly live in dry, desert areas and are active at night. They may be hiding under rocks, wood, or anything else lying on the ground. Some species may also burrow into the ground. To prevent scorpion stings, employees can wear long sleeves, pants, and leather gloves when practical. It is important to shake out shoes or clothing before donning. Additional information on first aid can be found at http://www.cdc.gov/niosh/topics/insects/.

Black widow spiders are commonly found in the southern and western areas of the United States. They are identified by the pattern of red coloration on the underside of their abdomen. They live in outdoor toilets where flies are plentiful or in undisturbed places such as under eaves and fences. A bite from a black widow can be distinguished by the two puncture marks it makes in the skin. The venom is a neurotoxin that produces pain at the bite area and then spreads to the chest, abdomen, or the entire body. Employees should inspect clothing, shoes, towels, or equipment before use, and wear clothing including long-sleeved shirt and long pants, hat, gloves, and boots when handling stacked or undisturbed piles of materials. Additional information on first aid can be found at http://www.cdc.gov/niosh/topics/spiders/.

Hantavirus Pulmonary Syndrome

Hantavirus pulmonary syndrome is a deadly disease transmitted by infected rodents through urine, droppings, or saliva [Mills et al. 2002]. In the southwestern United States, it is carried by deer mice and cotton and rice rats. Humans can contract the disease when they breathe in aerosolized virus. Rodent control in and around the workplace remains the primary strategy for preventing hantavirus infection. Additional information is available in the CDC documents, "Facts about Hantaviruses: What You Need to Know to Prevent the Disease Hantavirus Pulmonary Syndrome (HPS)" at http://www.cdc.gov/ncidod/dvrd/spb/mnpages/HPS_Brochure.pdf and "Hantavirus Pulmonary Syndrome (HPS): What You Need to Know" at http://www.cdc.gov/ncidod/diseases/hanta/hps/noframes/HPS_WhatYouNeedToKnow.pdf.

Hepatitis A

Hepatitis A is a contagious liver disease that results from infection with HAV. HAV is spread primarily by fecal/oral routes (often resulting from inadequate hand washing) and may be spread via contaminated food or water. Depending on environmental conditions, HAV can be stable in the environment for at least 30 days [McCaustland et al. 1982]. Since the 1960s, most hepatitis A cases have in occurred in the western and southwestern United States [Fiore et al. 2006]. Additional information on hepatitis A can be found at http://www.cdc.gov/hepatitis/A/PDFs/HepAGeneralFactSheet.pdf.

The data for the need for vaccinations for wastewater employees for HAV are mixed [Tooher et al. 2005]. Data from serologic studies conducted in Europe indicate that employees who had been exposed to sewage had a possible elevated risk for HAV infection [Poole and Shakespeare 1993; Lerman et al. 1999; Glas et al. 2001]. In published reports of three serologic surveys conducted among U.S. wastewater employees and appropriate comparison populations, no substantial or consistent increase in the prevalence of anti-HAV was identified among the employees [Trout et al. 2000; Weldon et al. 2000; Venczel 2003]. No cases of occupational HAV transmission among wastewater employees have been reported in the literature for the United States; however, there are isolated case reports for other countries including Canada [De Serres and Laliberté 1997]. The studies do not provide information about whether or not the employees were exposed to treated or untreated human waste.

Hepatitis B

Hepatitis B is a contagious liver disease caused by HBV. The disease can range in severity from a mild illness lasting a few weeks to a serious, lifelong illness. Hepatitis B is usually spread when blood, semen, or another body fluid from a person infected with the hepatitis B virus enters the body of someone who is not infected. This can happen through sexual contact with an infected person or sharing needles, syringes, or other drug-injection equipment. Hepatitis B can also be passed from an infected mother to her baby at birth. HBV can survive for at least 7 days outside the human body [Bond et al. 1981]. Vaccination is the best way to prevent hepatitis B. Additional information on hepatitis B can be found at http://www.cdc.gov/hepatitis/HBV/PDFs/HepBGeneralFactSheet.pdf.

References

ACGIH [2011]. 2010 TLVs® and BEIs®: threshold limit values for chemical substances and physical agents and biological exposure indices. Cincinnati, OH: American Conference of Governmental Industrial Hygienists.

AIHA [2010]. AIHA 2010 Emergency response planning guidelines (ERPG) & workplace environmental exposure levels (WEEL) handbook. Fairfax, VA: American Industrial Hygiene Association.

ATSDR [2004] Toxicological profile for ammonia. [http://www.atsdr.cdc.gov/toxprofiles/tp126.pdf]. Date accessed: June 2011.

Bond WW, Favero MS, Petersen NJ, Gravelle CR, Ebert JW, Maynard JE [1981]. Survival of hepatitis B virus after drying and storage for one week. Lancet 1(8219):550–551.

CFR. Code of Federal Regulations. Washington, DC: U.S. Government Printing Office, Office of the Federal Register.

De Serres G, Laliberté D [1997]. Hepatitis A among workers from a wastewater treatment plant during a small community outbreak. Occup Environ Med 54(1):60–62.

Glas C, Hotz P, Steffen R [2001]. Hepatitis A in workers exposed to sewage: a systematic review. Occup Environ Med 58(12):762–768.

Lerman Y, Chodick G, Aloni H, Ribak J, Ashkenazi S [1999]. Occupations at increased risk of hepatitis A: a 2-year nationwide historical prospective study. Am J Epidemiol 150(3):312–320.

McCaustland KA, Bond WW, Bradley DW, Ebert JW, Maynard JE [1982] Survival of hepatitis A virus in feces after drying and storage for 1 month. J Clin Microbiol 16(5):957–958.

Mills JN, Corneli A, Young JC, Garrison LE, Khan AS, Ksiazek TG [2002]. Hantavirus pulmonary syndrome – United States: updated recommendations for risk reduction. MMWR 51(RR-9):1–12.

NIOSH [2005]. NIOSH pocket guide to chemical hazards. Cincinnati, OH: U.S. Department of Health and Human Services, Centers for Disease Control and Prevention, National Institute for Occupational Safety and Health, DHHS (NIOSH) Publication No. 2005-149. [http://www.cdc.gov/niosh/npg/]. Date accessed: June 2011.

Poole CJ, Shakespeare AT [1993]. Should sewage workers and carers for people with learning disabilities be vaccinated for hepatitis A? Br Med J 306(6885):1102.

Tooher R, Griffin T, Shute E, Maddern G [2005]. Vaccinations for waste-handling workers. A review of the literature. Waste Manag Res 23(1):79–86.

Trout D, Mueller C, Venczel L, Krake A [2000]. Evaluation of occupational transmission of hepatitis A virus among wastewater workers. J Occup Environ Med 42(1):83–87.

Venczel L, Brown S, Frumkin H, Simmonds-Diaz J, Deitchman S, Bell BP [2003]. Prevalence of hepatitis A virus infection among sewage workers in Georgia. Am J Industrial Med 43(2):172–178.

Weldon M, VanEgdom MJ, Hendricks KA, Regner G, Bell BP, Sehulster LM [2000]. Prevalence of antibody to hepatitis A virus in drinking water workers and wastewater workers in Texas from 1996 to 1997. J Occup Environ Med 42(8):821–826.

APPENDIX B: CONFINED SPACE ENTRY REQUIREMENTS

Composting toilet vaults such as those described in this report meet NIOSH criteria for a confined space. NIOSH defines a confined space as "an area which by design has limited openings for entry and exit, unfavorable natural ventilation which could contain (or produce) dangerous air contaminant, and which is not intended for continuous employee occupancy" [NIOSH 1979]. The NIOSH criteria for working in confined spaces further classify confined spaces on the basis of the atmospheric characteristics such as oxygen level, flammability, and toxicity. As shown in Table B1, if any of the hazards present a situation that is IDLH, the confined space is designated Class A. A Class B confined space has the potential for causing injury and/or illness, but is not an IDLH atmosphere. A Class C confined space is one in which the hazard potential would not require any special modification of the work procedure. Table B2 lists the confined space program elements that are recommended (or must be considered by a qualified person, as defined by the criteria) before entering and during work within confined spaces on the basis of established hazard classification [29 CFR 1910.146]. The work in the composting toilets would be considered a Class C confined space.

Table B1. Confined space classification table [NIOSH 1979]

Parameters	Class A	Class B	Class C
Characteristics	IDLH* – rescue procedures require the entry of more than one individual fully equipped with life support equipment – maintenance of communication requires an additional standby person stationed within the confined space	Dangerous, but not immediately life threatening – rescue procedures require the entry of no more than one individual fully equipped with life support equipment – indirect visual or auditory communication with worker	Potential hazard – requires no modification of work procedures – standard rescue procedures – direct communication with workers, from outside the confined space
Oxygen	16% or less (122 mm Hg) or greater than 25% (190 mm HG)†	16.1% to 19.4% (122 – 147 mm Hg) or 21.5% to 25% (163 – 190 mm Hg)	19.5% – 21.4% (148 – 163 mm Hg)
Flammability Characteristics	20% or greater of LFL‡	10% – 19% LFL	10% LFL or less
Toxicity	IDLH	Greater than contamination level, referenced in 29 CFR Part 1910 Sub Part Z – less than IDLH	Less than contamination level referenced in 29 CFR Part 1910 Sub Part Z

*Immediately dangerous to life or health
†On the basis of a total atmospheric pressure of 760 millimeters of mercury (mm Hg) at sea level
‡Lower flammable limit

Table B2. NIOSH checklist of considerations for entry, working in, and exiting confined spaces [NIOSH 1979]

Item	Class A	Class B	Class C
1. Permit	X*	X	X
2. Atmospheric testing	X	X	X
3. Monitoring	X	O†	O
4. Medical surveillance	X	X	O
5. Training of personnel	X	X	X
6. Labeling and posting	X	X	X
7. Preparation			
Isolate/lockout/tag	X	X	O
Purge and ventilate	X	X	O
Cleaning processes	O	O	O
Requirements for special equipment/tools	X	X	O
8. Procedures			
Initial plan	X	X	X
Standby	X	X	O
Communications/observation	X	X	X
Rescue	X	X	X
Work	X	X	X
9. Safety equipment and clothing			
Head protection	O	O	O
Hearing protection	O	O	O
Hand protection	O	O	O
Foot protection	O	O	O
Body protection	O	O	O
Respiratory protection	O	O†	
Safety belts	X	X	X
Life lines, harness	X	O	
10. Rescue equipment	X	X	X
11. Record keeping/exposure	X	X	

*X—Indicates requirement
†O—Indicates determination by the qualified person

References

CFR. Code of Federal Regulations. Washington, DC: U.S. Government Printing Office, Federal Register.

NIOSH [1979]. Criteria for a recommended standard: working in confined spaces. Cincinnati, OH: U.S. Department of Health, Education, and Welfare, Center for Disease Control, National Institute for Occupational Safety and Health, DHEW (NIOSH).

ACKNOWLEDGMENTS AND AVAILABILITY OF REPORT

The Hazard Evaluations and Technical Assistance Branch (HETAB) of the National Institute for Occupational Safety and Health (NIOSH) conducts field investigations of possible health hazards in the workplace. These investigations are conducted under the authority of Section 20(a)(6) of the Occupational Safety and Health Act of 1970, 29 U.S.C. 669(a)(6) which authorizes the Secretary of Health and Human Services, following a written request from any employer or authorized representative of employees, to determine whether any substance normally found in the place of employment has potentially toxic effects in such concentrations as used or found. HETAB also provides, upon request, technical and consultative assistance to federal, state, and local agencies; labor; industry; and other groups or individuals to control occupational health hazards and to prevent related trauma and disease.

The findings and conclusions in this report are those of the authors and do not necessarily represent the views of NIOSH. Mention of any company or product does not constitute endorsement by NIOSH. In addition, citations to websites external to NIOSH do no constitute NIOSH endorsement of the sponsoring organizations or their programs or products. Furthermore, NIOSH is not responsible for the content of these websites. All Web addresses referenced in this document were accessible as of the publication date.

This report was prepared by Nancy Clark Burton and Chad Dowell of HETAB, Division of Surveillance, Hazard Evaluations and Field Studies. Analytical support was provided by Microbiology Specialists Inc., Houston, Texas. Health communication assistance was provided by Stefanie Evans. Editorial assistance was provided by Ellen Galloway. Desktop publishing was performed by Greg Hartle.

Copies of this report have been sent to employee and management representatives at the federal agency, the state health department, and the Occupational Safety and Health Administration Regional Office. This report is not copyrighted and may be freely reproduced. The report may be viewed and printed at http://www.cdc.gov/niosh/hhe/. Copies may be purchased from the National Technical Information Service (NTIS) at 5825 Port Royal Road, Springfield, Virginia 22161.

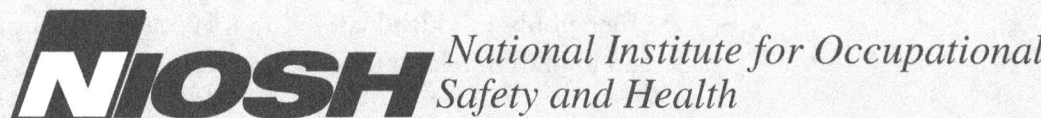 *National Institute for Occupational Safety and Health*

Delivering on the Nation's promise: Safety and health at work for all people through research and prevention.

To receive NIOSH documents or information about occupational safety and health topics, contact NIOSH at:

1-800-CDC-INFO (1-800-232-4636)

TTY: 1-888-232-6348

E-mail: cdcinfo@cdc.gov

or visit the NIOSH web site at: **www.cdc.gov/niosh.**

For a monthly update on news at NIOSH, subscribe to NIOSH eNews by visiting **www.cdc.gov/niosh/eNews.**

SAFER • HEALTHIER • PEOPLE™